PREFACE

My name is Valencia Annik Payne, BSN, RN, BS, Biology. I received my BS in Nursing from Delta State University and my BS in Biology from Jackson State University. I am a former Navy PACU RN that has instructed and tutored many nursing students, as well as, many Registered Nurses. As the Author of Fluid and Electrolytes for Nursing Students, now comes Dimensional Analysis for Nursing Students. A critical requirement of nursing is become math proficient. Learn how to safely administer medications and intravenous fluids. Also master mathematical competencies. This book provides colorful explanations and examples.

CONTENTS

DIMENSIONAL ANALYSIS

Dimensional analysis is a problem solving method that uses any expression or number that can be multiplied by one without changing its value.

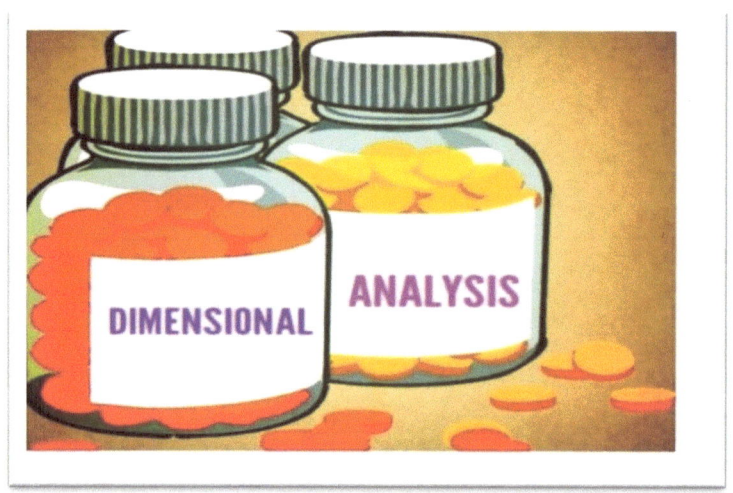

CONVERSION TABLE

1 gram = 1000 mg
1 mg = 1000 mcg
1 kg = 1000 grams
1 L = 1000 mL
1 kg = 2.2 lbs (pounds)
1 lbs = 16 oz (ounces)
1 oz = 30 mL
1 oz = 2 tablespoons
1 tablespoon = 15 mL
1 teaspoon = 5 mL

EXAMPLE PROBLEM: Your patient has Dilantin suspension 120 mg po t.i.d. ordered. In stock you have a bottle with liquid labeled Dilantin 75 mg/5mL. How much do you give in mL?

A. In order to solve any Med-Cal problem, always look for what the question is asking. In the example above you want to find **mL**.

B. When setting up your dimensional analysis solution, **ALWAYS WHAT YOU LOOK FOR GOES ON TOP!!**

C. **SET UP YOUR "FOOTBALL GOAL"!!**

$$\frac{5mL}{75mg} \left| \frac{120mg}{1} \right| = 8mL$$

PO PRACTICE PROBLEMS

1. Doctor's order: Coumadin 7.5 mg PO. Available is 5 mg-tablet. How many tablets will you administer to the client?

2. Doctor's order: Apresoline 25 mg. Available is Apresoline 50 mg/tablet. How many tablets will you administer to the client?

3. Doctor's order: Phenobarbital 90 mg. Available is Phenobarbital 30 mg/tablet. How many tablets will you administer to the patient?

4. Digoxin in a drug is used in connection with the heart. A stock bottle contains elixir with 0.05 mg/mL. If the prescription is 0.5 mg, how much elixir should be given to an adult?

5. A stock bottle of digoxin contains elixir with 0.05 mg/mL. If the prescription is 1 mg, how much elixir should be given?

6. The stock bottle of sulfadimidine, used to arrest the growth of bacteria, contains 75 mg/mL. The prescription reads 1500 mg as an initial dose. How many mL should be given orally?

7. A nurse takes the stock bottle of ampicillin 0.025 g/mL, to give an oral dose of 0.3 g. How many mL should be given?

8. A dosage of 400 mg is ordered. The solution strength is 250 mg in 2 mL. How many mL are required for this dose?

FLOW RATE

IV fluids maybe infused using an infusion pump or manual control. In order to calculate the flow rate, one must determine if the tubing to be used is a macrodrip or microdrip. The drip factor (also called the drop factor) is the number of drops per mL of solution delivered from the drip chamber.

A. Microdrip tubing delivers 60 gtt/mL. It is used to infuse precise and small amounts of fluids.

B. Macrodrip tubing delivers between 15 gtt/mL and 10 gtt/mL. It is used to infuse fluids rapidly and in large volumes.

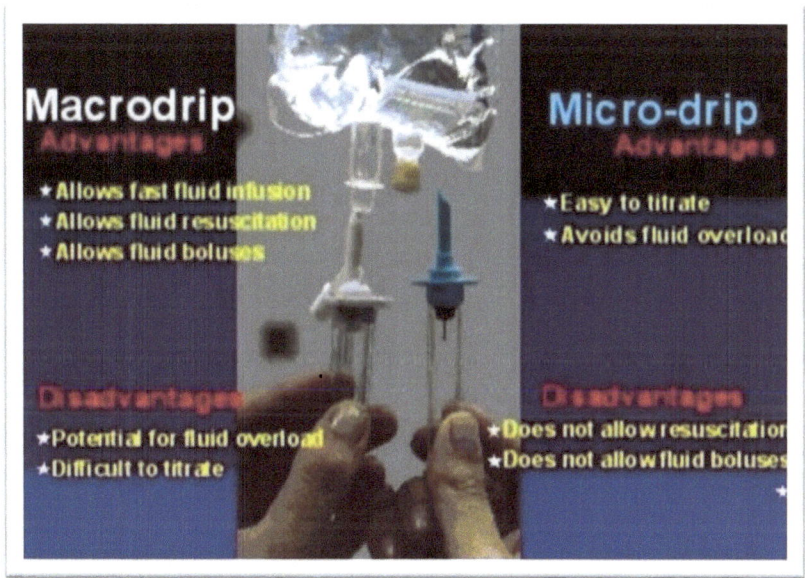

EXAMPLE PROBLEM: Prescribed is Medication B 200 mL to infuse over 90 min. The nurse should set the IV pump for how many mL/hr?

A. In order to solve any Med-Cal problem, always look for what the question is asking. In the example above you want to find **mL/hr**.

B. When setting up your dimensional analysis solution, ALWAYS WHAT YOU LOOK FOR GOES ON TOP!!

C. SET UP YOUR "FOOTBALL GOAL"!!

$$\frac{200\text{mL}}{90\text{min}} \left| \frac{60\text{min}}{1\text{hr}} \right. = 133\text{mL/hr}$$

FLOW RATE PRACTICE PROBLEMS

1. Infuse 1400 mL 0.45% NS in 16 hours. How many mL/hr will you set the IV pump to infuse?

2. Infuse Intralipid 20% 500 mL in 10 hours. How many mL/hr will you set the IV pump to infuse?

3. Infuse 1000 mL D5W in 6 hours. Drop factor is 20 gtt/mL. At what rate in gtt/min will the IV be regulated?

4. Infuse 1L NS in 10 hours. Drop factor is 20 gtt/mL. At what rate in gtt/min will the IV be regulated?

5. Ampicillin 1 g in 50 mL D5W to infuse over 45 minutes. Drop factor is 15 gtt/mL. At what rate in gtt/min will the IV be regulated?

6. Clindamycin 900 mg in 75 mL D5W over 30 minutes. Drop factor is 20 gtt/mL. At what rate in gtt/min will the IV regulated?

7. Doctor's order: Heparin 1700 Units/hour. Available: Heparin 25,000 in 500 mL 1/2 normal saline. What is the IV flow rate in mL/hr?

8. Doctor's order: Heparin 900 Units/hr. Available: Heparin 50,000 Units in 500 mL D5W. What is the flow rate in mL/hr?

IV INFUSION TIME

Understanding flow rates (mL/hr) is easy but what if you are given a problem on a test that will ask you how long (hours or minutes) it will take for an intravenous medication to infuse. In this section, you will practice and learn how long an infusion will last.

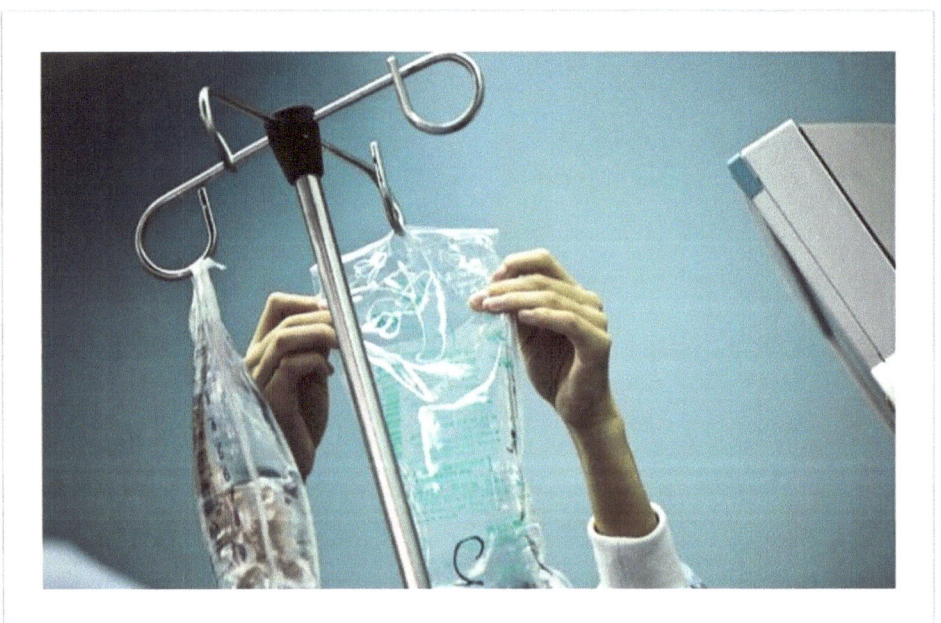

IV INFUSION TIME PRACTICE PROBLEMS

1. Your client will receive 2500mL of D5W with a flow rate of 150mL/hr. How long will it take to infuse?

2. Ampicillan 250mg IV in 100mL of NS to infuse over 45 minutes. How long will it take to infuse?

3. You receive an order for D5W 1000mL IV to infuse at 60mL/hr to begin at 0800. At what time will this IV be complete?

4. You receive an order for LR solution 1000mL IV to run at 130mL/hr. How long will this IV last?

INJECTION MEDICATIONS

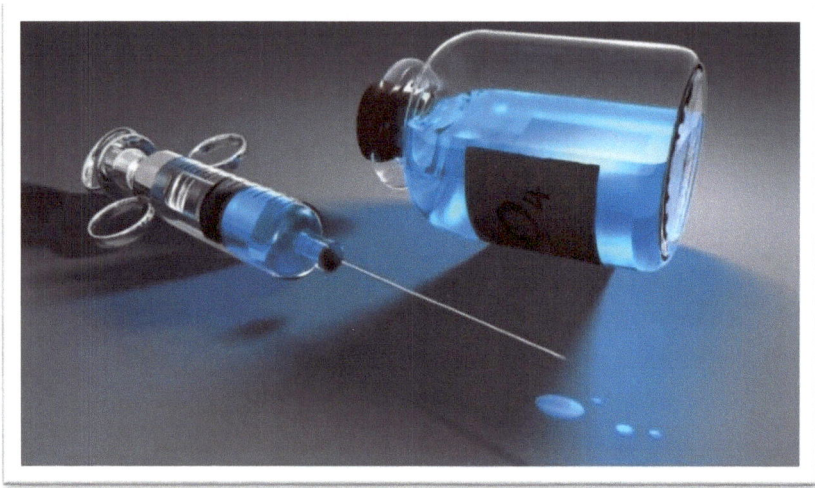

Injections are an infusion method of putting fluid into the body, usually with a syringe and a hollow needle which is pierced through the skin to a sufficient depth for the material to be administered into the body. **An injection follows a parenteral route which includes Intradermal, Subcutaneous, Intramuscular, and Intravenous**. The parenteral routes offer the reliable and direct method of administrating medications. It also provides the most rapid absorption. The disadvantages of using the parenteral route are tissue damage, pain and anxiety for the patient, and risk for infection.

EXAMPLE PROBLEM: A doctor orders Heparin 2500 Units. Heparin is available in 10,000 Units/mL. How many mL will you give?

A. In order to solve any Med-Cal problem, always look for what the question is asking. In the example above you want to find **mL**.

B. When setting up your dimensional analysis solution, ALWAYS WHAT YOU LOOK FOR GOES ON TOP!!

C. SET UP YOUR FOOTBALL GOAL!!

$$\frac{1\text{mL}}{10,000\text{ Units}} \cdot \frac{2500\text{ Units}}{1} = 0.25\text{mL}$$

INJECTION MEDICATION PRACTICE PROBLEMS

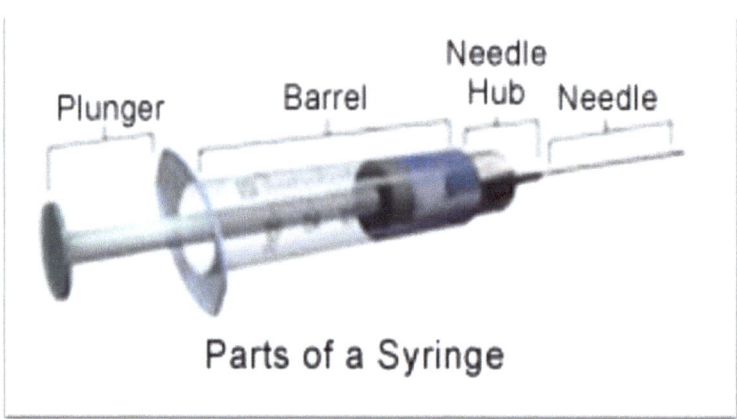

Parts of a Syringe

1. A doctor prescribes 30 mg of a drug to be given by injection. It is a drug dispensed in a solution of strength 60 mg/mL. How many mL should the health professional give?

2. A doctor prescribes 20 mg of a drug to be given by injection. It is a drug dispensed in a solution of strength 80 mg/mL. How many mL should the health professional give?

3. Morphine comes in 20 mg/mL. How many mL should be injected if 10 mg are prescribed?

4. How many mL should be injected if 15 mg of Morphine (20 mg/mL) are prescribed?

TYPES OF INJECTIONS

INTRADERMAL INJECTION

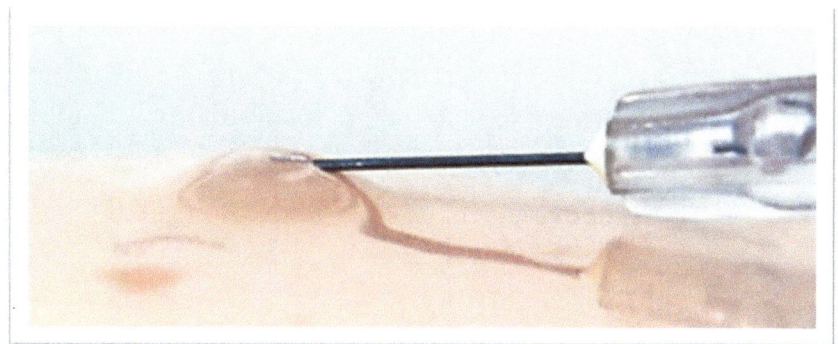

SUBCUTANEOUS INJECTION

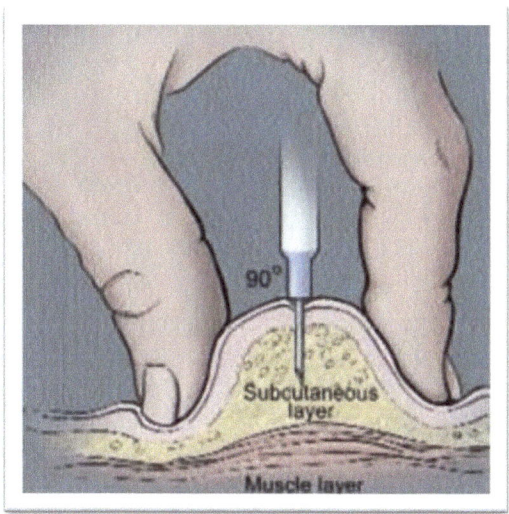

INTRAMUSCULAR INJECTION

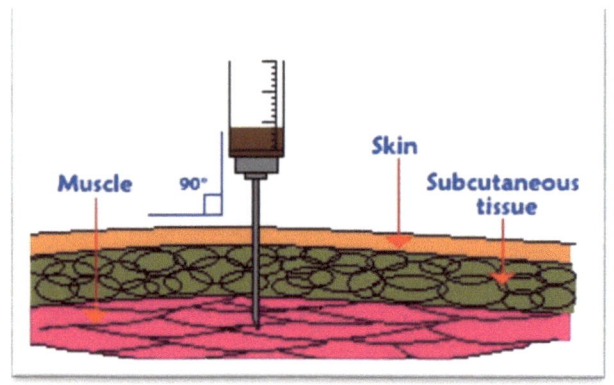

INTRAVENOUS

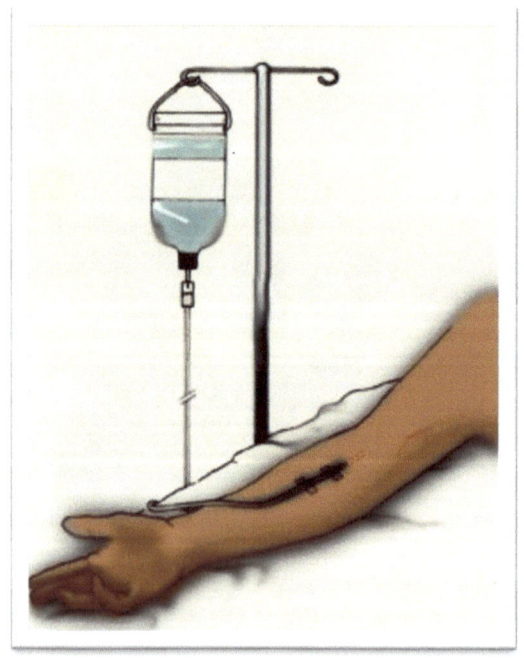

PO PRACTICE PROBLEM ANSWERS

1.

$$\frac{1\ tab}{5\ mg} \left| \frac{7.5\ mg}{1} \right| = 1.5\ tabs$$

2.

$$\frac{1\ tab}{50\ mg} \left| \frac{25\ mg}{1} \right| = 0.5\ tab$$

3.

$$\frac{1\ tab}{30\ mg} \left| \frac{90\ mg}{1} \right| = 3\ tabs$$

4.

$$\frac{1\ mL}{0.05\ mg} \left| \frac{0.5\ mg}{1} \right| = 10\ mL$$

5. $\dfrac{1\text{mL}}{0.05\text{mg}} \left| \dfrac{1\text{mg}}{1} \right| = 20\text{mg}$

6. $\dfrac{1\text{mL}}{75\text{mg}} \left| \dfrac{1500\text{mg}}{1} \right| = 20\text{mL}$

7. $\dfrac{1\text{mL}}{0.025\text{g}} \left| \dfrac{0.3\text{g}}{1} \right| = 12\text{mL}$

8. $\dfrac{2\text{mL}}{250\text{mg}} \left| \dfrac{400\text{mg}}{1} \right| = 3.2\text{mL}$

FLOW RATE PRACTICE PROBLEM ANSWERS

1.

$$\frac{1400mL}{16hrs} = 88mL/hr$$

2.

$$\frac{500mL}{10hr} = 50mL/hr$$

3.

$$\frac{20gtt}{1mL} \bigg| \frac{1000mL}{6hrs} \bigg| \frac{1hr}{60min} = 56gtt/min$$

4.

$$\frac{20gtt}{1mL} \bigg| \frac{1L}{10hrs} \bigg| \frac{1000mL}{1L} \bigg| \frac{1hr}{60min} =$$

$$33gtt/min$$

5.

$$\frac{15 gtt}{1 mL} \left| \frac{500 mL}{45 min} \right. = 17 gtt/min$$

6.

$$\frac{20 gtt}{1 mL} \left| \frac{75 mL}{30 min} \right. = 50 gtt/min$$

7.

$$\frac{500 mL}{25,000 units} \left| \frac{1700 units}{1 hr} \right. = 34 mL/hr$$

8.

$$\frac{500 mL}{50,000 units} \left| \frac{900 units}{1 hr} \right. = 9 mL/hr$$

IV INFUSION TIME PRACTICE PROBLEM ANSWERS

1.

$$\frac{1hr}{150mL} \mid \frac{2500mL}{1} \mid = 16.6 \text{ or } 17 hrs$$

2.

$$45min \mid \frac{1hr}{600min} \mid = 0.75hr$$

3.

$$\frac{1hr}{60mL} \mid \frac{1000mL}{1} \mid = 17hrs$$

It will be complete at 0100

4.

$$\frac{1\,hr}{130\,mL} \left| \frac{1000\,mL}{1} \right| = 8\,hrs$$

INJECTION MEDICATIONS PROBLEM ANSWERS

1.

$$\frac{1mL}{60mg} \cdot \frac{30mg}{1} = 0.5mL$$

2.

$$\frac{1mL}{80mg} \cdot \frac{20mg}{1} = 0.25mL$$

3.

$$\frac{1mL}{20mg} \cdot \frac{10mg}{1} = 0.5mL$$

4.

$$\frac{1mL}{20mg} \cdot \frac{15mg}{1} = 0.75mL$$

rn4students.net

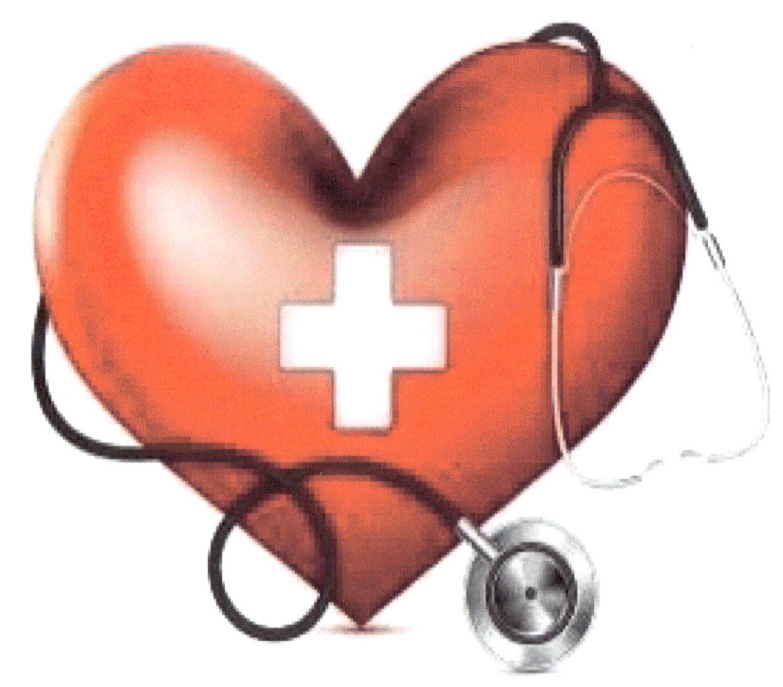

REFERENCE

Kee, J., & Marshall, S. (2004). Clinical calculations with applications to general and specialty areas. St. Louis, MO: Elsevier.

PHOTO CREDITS

http://www.pd4pic.com/pill/

http://coolwallpaperz.info/wallpaper/anime-fantasy-injection-d-widescreen-on-the-pictures-149168-wallpaper_w4950.html

http://www.firstcollege.ca/coming-up/medication-administration/

http://images.1233.tw/how-to-give-a-hormone-injection/

https://www.kyotokagaku.com/products/detail01/m94.html

http://www.fitnessuncovered.co.uk/article/how-to-inject-steroids

http://www.waiting.com/intravenous.html

http://www.tophealthmedical.com/syringes/

http://www.montessoricenter.org/academic-programs/summer-program/elementary-summer-program/

http://i.telegraph.co.uk/multimedia/archive/02931/Intravenous_drip_h_2931353b.jpg

www.ingramcontent.com/pod-product-compliance
Lightning Source LLC
Chambersburg PA
CBHW050428180526
45159CB00005B/2454

* 9 7 8 1 5 0 5 5 7 8 1 7 1 *